CW00459444

Lean And Green Cookbook 2021

A Self-Help Guide To Understanding Easy To Cook Recipes For Beginners To Transform Your Health And Radiate Vibrant Confidence For Quick Weight Loss And Lifelong Success

Lisa G. Torres

© Copyright 2021 - All rights reserved.

The content contained within this book may not be reproduced, duplicated or transmitted without direct written permission from the author or the publisher.

Under no circumstances will any blame or legal responsibility be held against the publisher, or author, for any damages, reparation, or monetary loss due to the information contained within this book. Either directly or indirectly.

Legal Notice:

This book is copyright protected. This book is only for personal use. You cannot amend, distribute, sell, use, quote or paraphrase any part, or the content within this book, without the consent of the author or publisher.

Disclaimer Notice:

Please note the information contained within this document is for educational and entertainment purposes only. All effort has been executed to present accurate, up to date, and reliable, complete information. No warranties of any kind are declared or implied. Readers acknowledge that the author is not engaging in the rendering of legal, financial, medical or professional advice. The content within this book has been derived from various sources. Please consult a licensed professional before attempting any techniques outlined in this book.

By reading this document, the reader agrees that under no circumstances is the author responsible for any losses, direct or indirect, which are incurred as a result of the use of information contained within this document, including, but not limited to, errors, omissions, or inaccuracies.

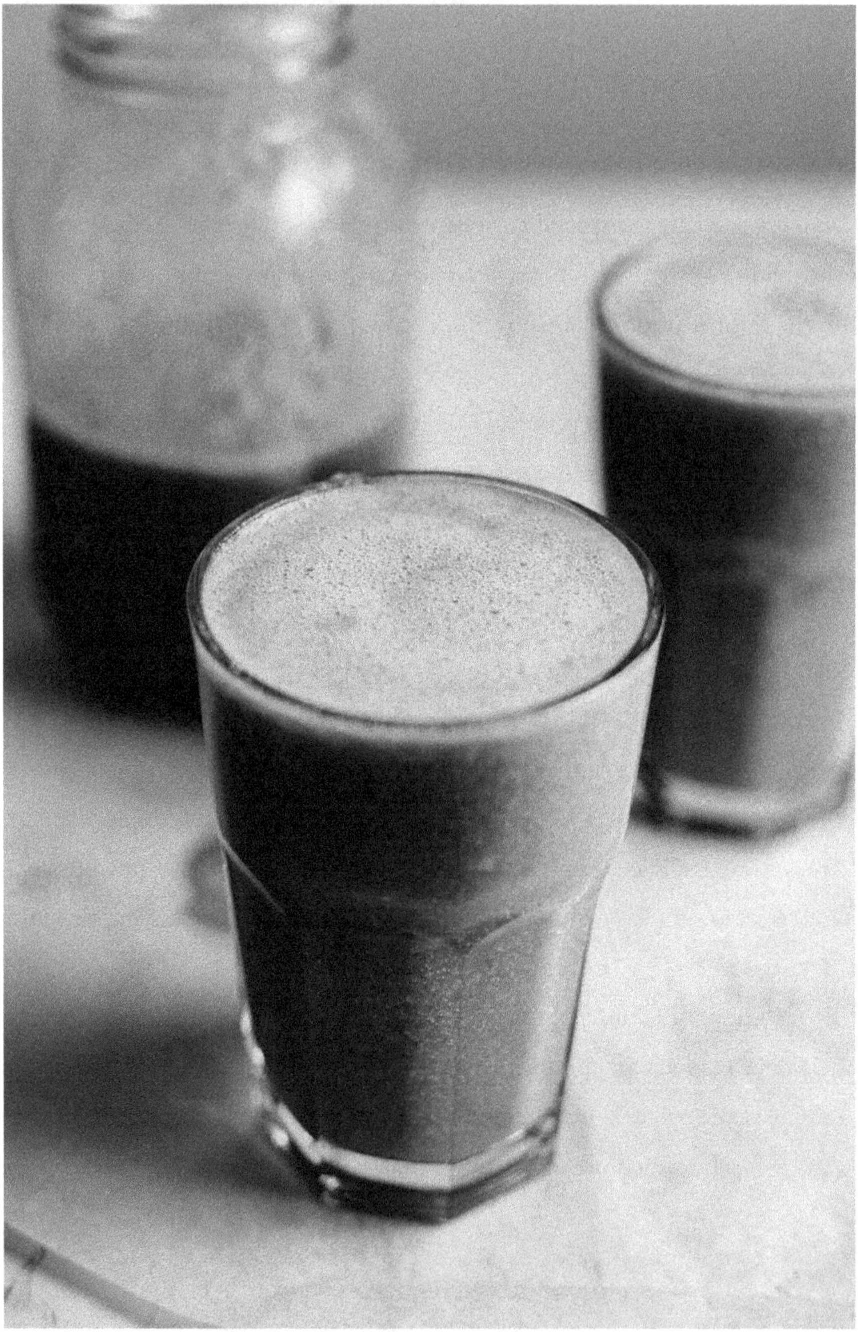

Table of Contents

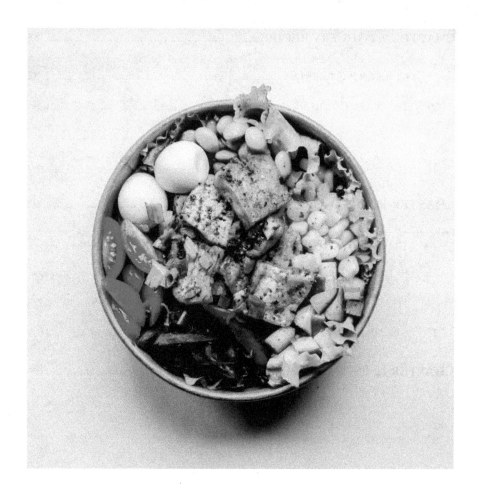

Introduction

If you are looking to lose weight fast and you don't always have enough time to cook, this regimen is the best option for you. However, this diet program requires that you work with a coach on a one-on-one guide and counseling. It includes branded products known as Fuelings and homemade food known as Lean & Green meals.

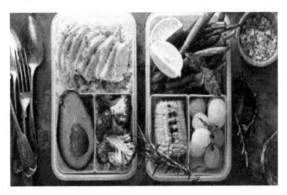

These Fuelings have over 60 products that are low in carb and high in protein. They have probiotic cultures with health-promoting bacteria that boost gut health. Some of them are bars, shakes, cereals, cookies, pasta, puddings, etc.

The Diet Programs

The program has three versions, which include 2 weight loss plans and a maintenance plan.

- **Optimal Weight 5&1**: This plan is the most popular among the program plans. It is made up of daily 5 Fuelings and 1 lean and green meal.

- **Optimal Weight 4&2&1**: If you need more calories, this plan is for you. It is more flexible and includes 4 Fuelings, 2 lean and green, and 1 snack every day.

- **Optimal Health 3&3**: With 3 Fuelings and 3 lean and green meals, it is designed to help in weight maintenance.

Diet Guide

For a quick weight loss goal, the Optimal Weight 5&1 Plan may be the best plan to start with. Most people with the target of losing weight usually go for this plan as it helps them to drop up to 12 pounds within 12 weeks.

In the Optimal Weight 5&1 Plan, you are expected to eat one lean and green meal and five Fuelings. These meals are to be eaten every 2-3 hours intervals. Then, you will back it up with 30 minutes of exercise. Your coach will direct you on the best approach.

However, the daily carbs from meals and Fuelings should not exceed 100 grams. You can get meals and Fuelings from the company. Though it may not be cost-effective, this book is designed to help you save costs. You can prepare the meals by yourself to reduce costs.

There are a plethora of recipes in this book to help you along the process for your daily meals. You can also eat out, but keep in mind that you must follow the diet plan as instructed by your coach. However, alcohol is highly restricted for this plan.

Once you get to your desired weight, you are expected to enter the maintenance phase. This is a transition phase that requires a gradual increase in your daily calorie intake to no more than 1,550 cal. You can add a wider variety of food to your daily meals, which include fruits, whole grains, and low-fat dairy.

The maintenance phase is expected to last for 6 weeks before you move to the Optimal Health 3&3 Plan. In this plan, your daily food intake will be 3 Fuelings and 3 lean and green meals.

In this diet, most people that follow the diet usually opt for the 5&1 plan. The 5&1 program is made up of 5 Fuelings and 1 high protein low-carb meal. There are over 60 fueling options in this diet, and these options include bars, puddings, shakes, soups, biscuits, etc. These Fuelings contain probiotics that help to promote digestive health.

The interesting aspect of this diet is its flexibility, which makes it easier to work with. Once you reach your desired weight goal, you can easily switch to the 3&3 plan. Transitioning to this weight-maintenance plan is easy since you have already changed the old unhealthy eating habits. For those looking to consume more calories, the 4&2&1 plan is your best bet. With the 4&2&1 plan, you take 4 Fuelings, 2 healthy lean and green meals, and 1 snack.

How This Diet Can Help You Lose Weight

How much weight you lose on the this diet depends mostly on how active and how you follow the plan. If you stick with the plan and stay very active, you will lose more weight. Many have tried it, and it worked perfectly well. The following research studies show how effective the diet can be when strictly followed. Though the research is mostly on Medifast, this diet and Medifast have identical macro-nutrients and can be interchanged to achieve the same result. So, the studies are valid for both this diet and Medifast plans.

- A study published in the Obesity journal in 2016 showed that after 12 weeks of observing the diet guides, obese people lost 8.8% body weight.

- The study released by John Hopkins Medicine that ran for 12 weeks revealed that weight-loss programs like Medifast are effective for a long-term weight loss goal.

- A study in the Nutrition Journal carried out in 2015 shows that 310 obese and overweight people who followed the diet plans lost 24 lb in 12 weeks. In the 24th week, the average weight loss recorded was 35 lb.

- Another study published in the Nutrition Journal shows that 90 obese adults who followed the 5&1 plan lost an average of 30 pounds in 16 weeks.

- The analysis published in the Eating and Weight Disorder Journal in 2008 shows that the average weight loss recorded on

324 obese patients in 12 weeks was 21 lb and 26 ½ lb after 24 weeks. However, these patients also took appetite suppressant.

Is Diet Easy To Follow?

If you are someone like me that likes trying so many treats and yummy recipes almost every day, the present regimen may not be easy in the long term. However, this diet is programmed to accommodate both long-term and short-term goals. There are three major diet plans to choose from to suit your desired eating habit.

The 5&1 plan may not be easy in the long-term, but there are over 60 fueling options to work with. Moreover, you have a plethora of resources where you can get recipes, including this cookbook with so many mouthwatering recipes to make.

Unlike most weight-loss diets, you don't need to stress yourself counting calories, points, or carbs. Though they are needed for reference purposes, you don't need to kill yourself over it as long as the meals you are taking are lean and green meals.

Interestingly, you can easily eat out while on this diet. The main thing is for you to understand the guidelines and follow them judiciously. You can as well download the eating out guide from the company website to help you easily navigate the buffets and eateries.

CHAPTER 1:

What to Eat

Best Foods for LEAN and GREEN Diet

Your homemade meals are expected to be mostly low-carb vegetables, lean proteins, and a few healthy fats. Low-carb beverages such as coffee, water, tea, unsweetened almond milk, etc, are allowed, but in small amounts.

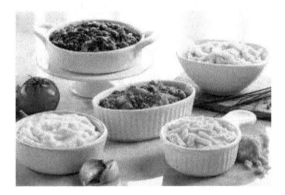

- The recommended foods for your lean and green meals are;

- Fish and Shellfish: trout, halibut, salmon, shrimp, tuna, crab, lobster, scallops.

- Meat: Lean beef, pork chop, tenderloin, turkey, chicken, lamb.

- Eggs: egg whites, whole eggs, and egg beaters.

- Soy: tofu

- Oil: vegetable oils - flaxseed, olive, canola, walnut, lemon oil, etc

- Fats: avocado, olives, almonds, pistachios, reduced-fat margarine, walnuts, etc.

- Vegetables: zucchini, cauliflower, celery, mushrooms, eggplant, pepper, spinach, cucumbers, squash, broccoli, collard, jicama, etc.

- Snacks (sugar-free): mints, popsicle, gum, gelatin, etc.

- Beverages (sugar-free): coffee, water, tea, almond milk, etc.

- Seasoning and condiments: spices, dried herbs, salsa, cocktail sauce, yellow mustard, lemon juice, soy sauce, lime juice, etc.

Avoid These Foods

Except for the carbs in the Fuelings, the present diet restricts most foods and beverages with carb content. Some fats are not allowed, including fried foods. Avoid the following foods in your daily meals;

- Refined grains: including pasta, flour tortillas, cookies, white rice, white bread, cakes, biscuits, etc.

- Whole fat dairy: including yogurt, milk, and cheese.

- Fried foods: including fish, veggies, meats, pastries, etc.

- Fats: like coconut oil, butter, etc.

- Alcohol: all types.

- Beverages: like an energy drink, fruit juice, sweet tea, soda, etc

If you are on the 5&1 plan, you need to avoid the following foods in your daily meal. You can introduce them in the transition phase;

- Starchy veggies: white potatoes, sweet potatoes, peas, and corn.

- Whole grains: brown rice, whole grain bread, whole-wheat pasta, etc.

- Low-fat dairy: cheese, yogurt, and milk.

- Legumes: beans, peas, soybeans, lentils, etc.

- Fruits: fresh fruits. Eat more berries when you enter the transition phase.

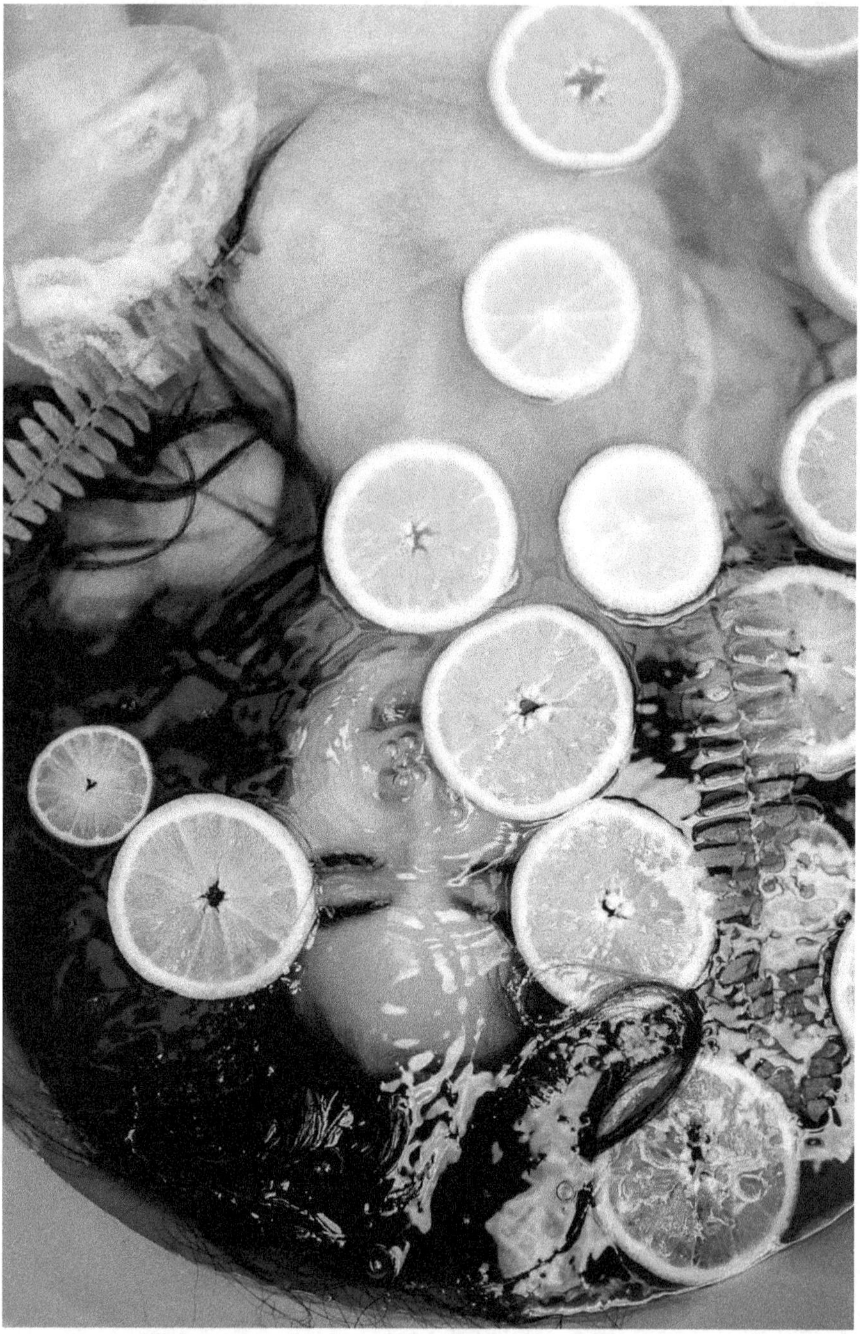

CHAPTER 2:

Lean and Green Recipes

1.   Savory Cilantro Salmon

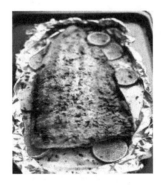

Preparation Time: 10 minutes

Cooking Time: 30 minutes

Servings: 4

Ingredients:

- 2 tablespoons of fresh lime or lemon

- 4 cups of fresh cilantro, divided

- 2 tablespoon of hot red pepper sauce

- ½ teaspoon of salt. Divided

- 1 teaspoon of cumin

- 4, 7 oz. of salmon filets

- ½ cup of (4 oz.) water

- 2 cups of sliced red bell pepper

- 2 cups of sliced yellow bell pepper

- 2 cups of sliced green bell pepper

- Cooking spray

- ½ teaspoon of pepper

Directions:

1. Get a blender or food processor and combine half of the cilantro, lime juice or lemon, cumin, hot red pepper sauce, water, and salt; then puree until they become smooth. Transfer the marinade gotten into a large re-sealable plastic bag.

2. Add salmon to marinade. Seal the bag, squeeze out air that might have been trapped inside, turn to coat salmon. Refrigerate for about 1 hour, turning as often as possible.

3. Now, after marinating, preheat your oven to about 400°F. Arrange the pepper slices in a single layer in a slightly-greased, medium-sized square baking dish. Bake it for 20 minutes, turn the pepper slices once.

4. Drain your salmon and do away with the marinade. Crust the upper part of the salmon with the remaining chopped, fresh cilantro.

5. Place salmon on the top of the pepper slices and bake for about 12-14 minutes until you observe that the fish flakes easily when it is being tested with a fork

6. Enjoy

Nutrition: Calories 350, Fat 13, Carbs 15, Protein 42

2.   Lean and Green "Macaroni"

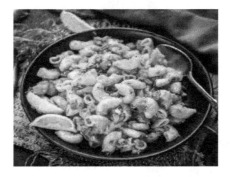

Preparation Time: 10 minutes

Cooking Time: 30 minutes

Servings: 2

Ingredients

- 2 tablespoons yellow onion, diced

- 5 ounces 95-97% lean ground beef

- 2 tablespoons light thousand island dressing

- 1/8 teaspoon apple cider vinegar

- 1/8 teaspoon onion powder

- 3 cups Romaine lettuce, shredded

- 2 tablespoons low-fat cheddar cheese, shredded

- 1-ounce dill pickle slices

- 1 teaspoon sesame seeds

Directions:

1. Put 3 tablespoons of water in a pan and heat over medium-low flame. Water sauté the onions for 30 seconds before adding the beef. Sauté the beef for 4 minutes while stirring constantly.

2. Add in the thousand island dressing, apple cider vinegar, and onion powder. Close the lid and keep on cooking for 5 minutes.

Remove the lid and allow to simmer until the sauce thickens.

Turn off the heat and allow the beef to rest and cool.

3. In a bowl, place the lettuce at the bottom and pour in the beef.

   Layer with cheddar cheese and pickles. Sprinkle with sesame on

   top.

Nutrition: Calories 412, Fat 8, Carbs 18, Protein 4

3.   Lean and Green Broccoli Taco

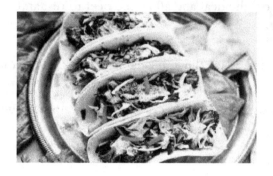

Preparation Time: 10 minutes

Cooking Time: 15 minutes

Servings: 2

Ingredients:

- 4 ounces 95-97% lean ground beef

- ¼ cup roma tomatoes, chopped

- ¼ teaspoon garlic powder

- ¼ teaspoon onion powder

- 1 ¼ cup broccoli, cut into bite-sized pieces

- A pinch of red pepper flakes

- 1 ounce low-sodium cheddar cheese, shredded

Directions:

1. Place 3 tablespoons of water in a pan and heat over medium flame. Water sauté the beef and tomatoes for 5 minutes until the tomatoes are wilted. Add in the garlic and onion powder and stir for another 3 minutes.

2. Add the broccoli and close the lid. Cook for another 5 minutes.

3. Garnish with red pepper flakes and cheddar cheese on top.

Nutrition: Calories 412, Fat 6, Carbs 20, Protein 6

4.   Lean and Green Crunchy Chicken Tacos

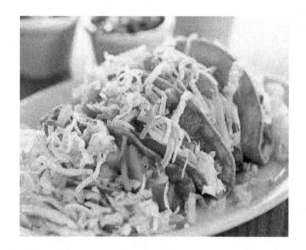

Preparation Time: 10 minutes

Cooking Time: 10 minutes

Servings: 2

Ingredients:

- ½ cup low sodium chicken stock

- 2 chicken breasts, minced

- 1 red onion, chopped

- 1 clove of garlic, minced

- 3 plum tomatoes, chopped

- 1 teaspoon cumin powder 1 teaspoon cinnamon powder

- 1 teaspoon ground coriander

- 1 red onion, chopped ½ red chili, chopped

- 1 tablespoon lime juice Meat from 1 ripe avocado

- 1 cucumber, sliced into thick rounds

Directions:

1. Place a tablespoon of chicken stock in a pan and heat over medium flame. Water sauté the chicken, onion, garlic, and tomatoes for 4 minutes or until the tomatoes have wilted.

2. Season with cumin, cinnamon, and coriander. Reduce the heat to low and cook for another 5 minutes. Set aside and allow to cool.

3. In a bowl, mix together the onion, chili, lime juice, and mashed avocado. This is the salsa.

4. Scoop the salsa and top on sliced cucumber. Top with cooked chicken.

Nutrition: Calories 447, Fat 8, Carbs 12, Protein 24

CHAPTER 3:

Fuelings

5.   Avocado Cream

Preparation time: 10 minutes

Cooking time: 10 minutes

Servings: 4

Ingredients:

- 2 avocados, pitted, peeled, and chopped

- 1 cup almond milk

- 2 scallions, chopped

- Salt and black pepper to the taste

- 2 tablespoons coconut oil

- 1 tablespoon chives, chopped

Directions:

1. Heat up a pot with the coconut oil over medium heat.

2. Add scallions and avocado and cook for 2 minutes.

Nutrition: calories 162, fat 4.4, carbs 6, protein 6

6.   Spicy kale chips

Prep time: 10 min

Cooking time: 30 min

Serving: 2

Ingredients:

- 1 large head of curly kale, wash, dry, and pulled from stem 1 tbsp extra virgin olive oil

- Minced parsley

- Squeeze of lemon juice

- Cayenne pepper

- Dash of soy sauce

Directions:

1. In a large bowl, rip the kale from the stem into palm-sized pieces.

2. Sprinkle the minced parsley, olive oil, soy sauce, a squeeze lemon juice, and a very small pinch of the cayenne powder.

3. Toss with a set of tongs or salad forks, and make sure to coat all of the leaves.

4. If you have a dehydrator, turn it on to 118F, spread out the kale on a dehydrator sheet, and leave it there for about 2 hours.

5. If you are cooking them, place parchment paper on top of a cookie sheet.

6. Lay the bed of kale and separate it a bit to make sure the kale is evenly toasted.

7. Cook for 10-15 minutes maximum at 250F.

Nutrition: Calories 284, Fat 5, Carbs 16, Protein 21

7.   Sweet and Savory Guacamole

Preparation time: 10 minutes

Cooking time: 15 minutes

Serving: 2

Ingredients:

- 2 large avocados, pitted and scooped

- 2 Medjool dates, pitted and sliced into pieces

- ½ cup cherry tomatoes, cut into halves

- 5 sprigs of parsley, chopped

- ¼ cup of arugula, chopped

- 5 sticks of celery, washed, cut into sticks for dipping

- Juice from ¼ lime

- Dash of sea salt

Directions:

1. Mash the avocado in a bowl, sprinkle salt, and squeeze lime juice.

2. Fold in the tomatoes, dates, herbs, and greens.

3. Scoop with celery sticks, and enjoy!

Nutrition: Calories 233, Fat 2, Carbs 2, Protein 6

8. Mushroom Scramble Eggs

Preparation time: 5 minutes

Cooking time: 30 minutes

Serving: 2

Ingredients:

- 2 eggs

- 1 tsp ground turmeric

- 1 tsp mellow curry powder

- 20g kale, generally slashed

- 1 tsp additional virgin olive oil

- ½ superior bean stew, daintily cut

- A bunch of catch mushrooms, meagerly cut

- 5g parsley, finely slashed

Directions:

1. Blend the turmeric and curry powder and include a little water until you have accomplished a light glue.

2. Steam the kale for 2-3 minutes.

3. Warmth the oil in a skillet over medium heat and fry the bean stew and mushrooms for 2-3 minutes until they have begun to darker and mollify.

4. Include the eggs and flavor glue and cook over a medium warmth, at that point add the kale and keep on cooking over medium heat for a further moment. At long last, include the parsley, blend well and serve.

Nutrition: Calories 324, Fat 3, Carbs 10, Protein 23

CHAPTER 4:

Lunch Recipes

9. Beef Curry

Preparation time: 15 minutes

Cooking time: 2¼ hours

Servings: 8

Ingredients

- 2 tablespoons olive oil

- 1 small yellow onion, chopped

- 1 green bell pepper, seeded and chopped

- 4 garlic cloves, minced

- 1 jalapeño pepper, chopped

- 1 teaspoon dried thyme, crushed

- 2 tablespoons red chili powder

- 1 tablespoon ground cumin

- 2 pounds lean ground turkey

- 2 cups fresh tomatoes, chopped finely

- 2 ounces sugar-free tomato paste

- 2 cups homemade chicken broth

- 1 cup water

- Salt and ground black pepper, as required

- 1 cup cheddar cheese, shredded

Directions:

1. In a large Dutch oven, heat oil over medium heat and sauté the onion and bell pepper for about 5–7 minutes.

2. Add the garlic, jalapeño pepper, thyme, and spices and sauté for about 1 minute.

3. Add the turkey and cook for about 4–5 minutes.

4. Stir in the tomatoes, tomato paste, and cacao powder, and cook for about 2 minutes.

5. Add in the broth and water and bring to a boil.

6. Now, reduce the heat to low and simmer, covered for about 2 hours.

7. Add in salt and black pepper and remove from the heat.

8. Top with cheddar cheese and serve hot.

Nutrition: Calories 234, Fat 12, Carbs 4, Protein 24

10.   Shepherd's pie

Preparation time: 20 minutes

Cooking time: 50 minutes

Servings: 6

Ingredients:

- ¼ cup olive oil

- 1 pound grass-fed ground beef

- ½ cup celery, chopped

- ¼ cup yellow onion, chopped

- 3 garlic cloves, minced

- 1 cup tomatoes, chopped

- 2 (12-ounce) packages riced cauliflower, cooked and well drained

- 1 cup cheddar cheese, shredded

- ¼ cup Parmesan cheese, shredded

- 1 cup heavy cream

- 1 teaspoon dried thyme

Directions:

1. Preheat your oven to 350°F.

2. Heat oil in a large nonstick wok over medium heat and cook the ground beef, celery, onions, and garlic for about 8–10 minutes.

3. Remove from the heat and drain the excess grease.

4. Immediately stir in the tomatoes.

5. Transfer mixture into a 10x7-inch casserole dish evenly.

6. In a food processor, add the cauliflower, cheeses, cream, and thyme, and pulse until a mashed potatoes-like mixture is formed.

7. Spread the cauliflower mixture over the meat in the casserole dish evenly.

8. Bake for about 35–40 minutes.

9. Remove casserole dish from oven and let it cool slightly before serving.

10. Cut into desired sized pieces and serve.

Nutrition: Calories 404, Fat 5, Carbs 9, Protein 23

11. Meatballs Curry

Preparation time: 15 minutes

Cooking time: 25 minutes

Servings: 6

Meatballs

- 1 pound lean ground pork

- 2 organic eggs, beaten

- 3 tablespoons yellow onion, finely chopped

- ¼ cup fresh parsley leaves, chopped

- ¼ teaspoon fresh ginger, minced

- 2 garlic cloves, minced

- 1 jalapeño pepper, seeded and finely chopped

- 1 teaspoon granulated erythritol

- 1 teaspoon curry powder

- 3 tablespoons olive oil

Curry

- 1 yellow onion, chopped

- Salt, as required

- 2 garlic cloves, minced

- ¼ teaspoon fresh ginger, minced

- 1 tablespoon curry powder

- 1 (14-ounce) can unsweetened coconut milk

- Ground black pepper, as required

- ¼ cup fresh parsley, minced

Directions:

For meatballs:

1. Place all the ingredients (except oil) in a large bowl and mix until well combined.

2. Make small-sized balls from the mixture.

3. Heat the oil in a large wok over medium heat and cook meatballs for about 3–5 minutes or until golden-brown from all sides.

4. Transfer the meatballs into a bowl.

For curry:

5. In the same wok, add onion and a pinch of salt, and sauté for about 4–5 minutes.

6. Add the garlic and ginger, and sauté for about 1 minute.

7. Add the curry powder and sauté for about 1–2 minutes.

8. Add coconut milk and meatballs, and bring to a gentle simmer.

9. Adjust the heat to low and simmer, covered for about 10–12 minutes.

10. Season with salt and black pepper and remove from the heat.

11. Top with parsley and serve.

Nutrition: Calories 350, Fat 13, Carbs 6, Protein 16

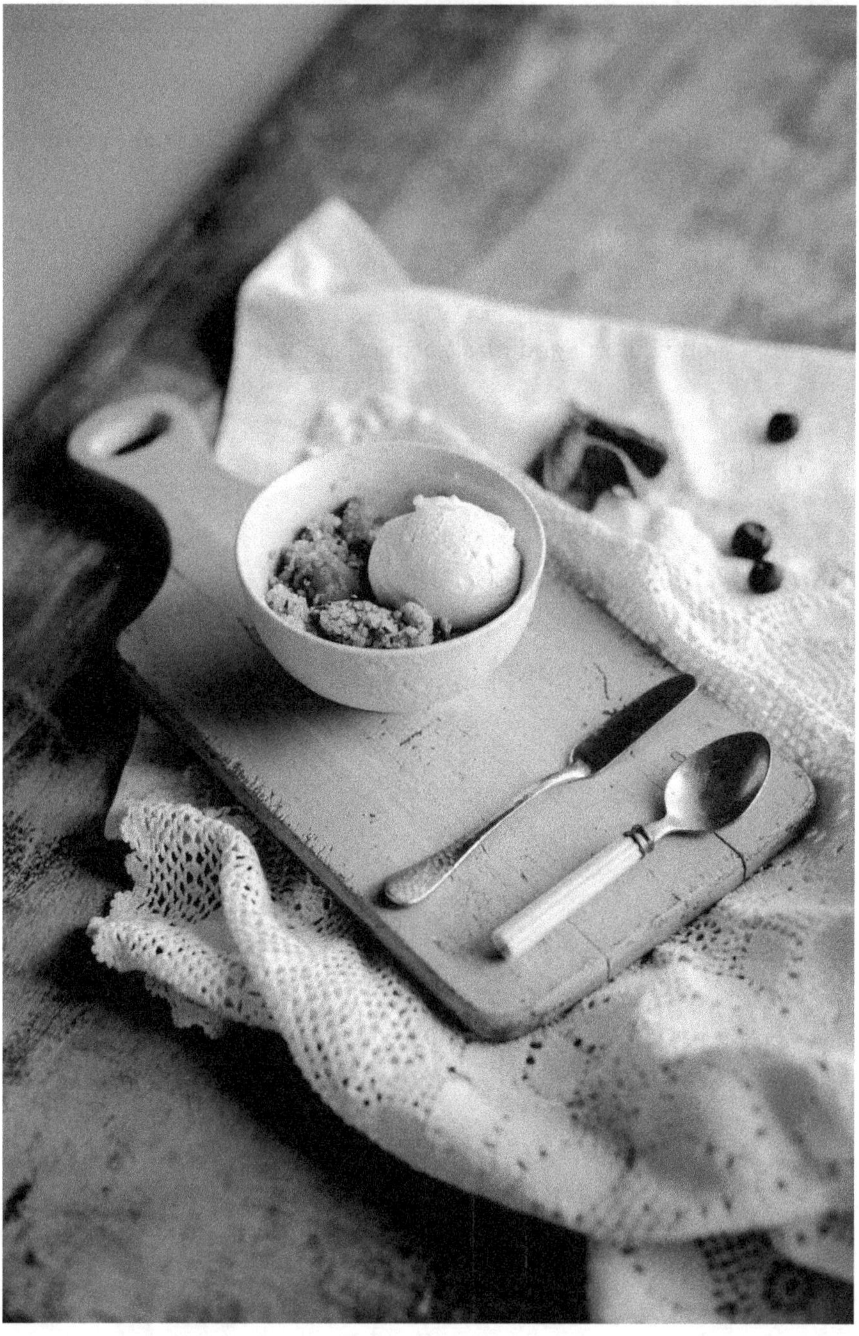

CHAPTER 5:

Dinner Recipes

12.   Steak and Mushroom Noodles

Preparation time: 10 minutes Cooking time: 20 minutes

Servings: 4

Ingredients:

- 100g shitake mushrooms, halved, if large

- 100g chestnut mushrooms, sliced

- 150g udon noodles

- 75g kale, finely chopped

- 75g baby leaf spinach, chopped

- 2 sirloin steaks

- 2 teaspoons miso paste

- 2.5cm piece fresh ginger, finely chopped

- 1 star anise 1 red chili, finely sliced

- 1 red onion, finely chopped

- 1 fresh coriander (cilantro) chopped

- 1 liter (1½ pints) warm water

Directions:

1. Pour the water into a saucepan and add in the miso, star anise, and ginger. Bring it to the boil, reduce the heat, and simmer

gently. In the meantime, cook the noodles according to their instructions, then drain them.

2. Heat the oil in a saucepan, add the steak and cook for around 2-3 minutes on each side (or 1-2 minutes, for rare meat).

3. Remove the meat and set aside.

4. Place the mushrooms, spinach, coriander (cilantro), and kale into the miso broth and cook for 5 minutes.

5. In the meantime, heat the remaining oil in a separate pan and fry the chili and onion for 4 minutes, until softened.

6. Serve the noodles into bowls and pour the soup on top.

7. Thinly slice the steaks and add them to the top. Serve immediately.

Nutrition: calories: 296, carbs: 24, Fat: 13, Protein: 32

13. Masala Scallops

Preparation time: 10 minutes

Cooking time: 20 minutes

Servings: 4

Ingredients:

- 2 jalapenos, chopped

- 1 pound sea scallops

- A pinch of salt and black pepper

- ¼ teaspoon cinnamon powder

- 1 teaspoon garam masala

- 1 teaspoon coriander, ground

- 1 teaspoon cumin, ground

- 2 tablespoons cilantro, chopped

Directions:

1. Heat up a pan with the oil over medium heat, add the jalapenos, cinnamon, and the other ingredients except for the scallops and cook for 10 minutes.

Nutrition: Calories: 251, Fat: 4g, Carbs: 11g, Protein: 17g

14.   Tuna and Tomatoes

Preparation time: 5 minutes

Cooking time: 20 minutes

Servings: 4

Ingredients:

- 1 yellow onion, chopped 1 tablespoon olive oil

- 1 cup tomatoes, chopped

- 1 red pepper, chopped 1 teaspoon sweet paprika

- 1 tablespoon coriander, chopped

Directions:

1. Heat up a pan with the oil over medium heat, add the onions and the pepper and cook for 5 minutes.

2. Add the fish and the other ingredients, cook everything for 15 minutes, divide between plates and serve.

Nutrition: Calories: 215, Fat: 4g, Carbs: 14g, Protein: 7g

15.   Lemongrass and Ginger Mackerel

Preparation: 10 minutes Cooking: 25 minutes Servings: 4

Ingredients:

- 4 mackerel fillets, skinless and boneless

- 1 tablespoon ginger, grated

- 2 lemongrass sticks, chopped

- 2 red chilies, chopped

- Juice of 1 lime A handful parsley, chopped

Directions:

1. In a roasting pan, combine the mackerel with the oil, ginger, and the other ingredients, toss and bake at 390 degrees F for 25 minutes.

2. Divide everything between plates and serve.

Nutrition: Calories: 251, Fat: 3, Carbs: 14, Protein: 8

16.   Scallops with Almonds and Mushrooms

Preparation time: 5 minutes **Cooking time:** 10 minutes

Servings: 4

Ingredients:

- 1 pound scallops 4 scallions, chopped

- A pinch of salt and black pepper

- ½ cup mushrooms, sliced

- 2 tablespoon almonds, chopped 1 cup coconut cream

Directions:

1. Heat up a pan with the oil over medium heat, add the scallions and the mushrooms and sauté for 2 minutes.

Nutrition: Calories: 322, Fat: 23.7, Carbs: 8.1, Protein: 21.6

CHAPTER 6:

Soup and Salads

17.   Cauliflower Spinach Soup

Preparation time: 45 minutes **Cooking time:** 25 minutes

Servings: 5

Ingredients:

- 1/2 cup unsweetened coconut milk

- 5 oz fresh spinach, chopped

- 5 watercress, chopped

- 8 cups vegetable stock

- 1 lb cauliflower, chopped

- Salt

Directions:

1. Add stock and cauliflower in a large saucepan and bring to a boil over medium heat for 15 minutes.

2. Add spinach and watercress and cook for another 10 minutes.

3. Remove from heat and puree the soup using a blender until smooth.

4. Add coconut milk and stir well. Season with salt.

5. Stir well and serve hot.

Nutrition: calories 150, fat 4, carbs 8, protein 11

18.   Avocado Mint Soup

Preparation time: 10 minutes

Cooking time: 10 minutes

Servings: 2

Ingredients:

- 1 medium avocado, peeled, pitted, and cut into pieces

- 1 cup coconut milk

- 2 romaine lettuce leaves 20 fresh mint leaves

- 1 tbsp fresh lime juice 1/8 tsp salt

Directions:

1. Add all ingredients into the blender and blend until smooth. The soup should be thick, not as a puree.

2. Pour into the serving bowls and place in the refrigerator for 10

   minutes.

3. Stir well and serve chilled.

Nutrition: calories 290, fat 3, carbs 18, protein 11

19.   Creamy Squash Soup

Preparation time: 35 minutes

Cooking time: 22 minutes

Servings: 8

Ingredients:

- 3 cups butternut squash, chopped

- 1 ½ cups unsweetened coconut milk

- 1 tbsp coconut oil

- 1 tsp dried onion flakes

- 1 tbsp curry powder

- 4 cups water

- 1 garlic clove

- 1 tsp kosher salt

Directions:

1. Add squash, coconut oil, onion flakes, curry powder, water, garlic, and salt into a large saucepan. Bring to a boil over high heat.

2. Turn heat to medium and simmer for 20 minutes.

3. Puree the soup using a blender until smooth. Return soup to the saucepan and stir in coconut milk and cook for 2 minutes.

4. Stir well and serve hot.

Nutrition: calories 140, fat 2, carbs 9, protein 1

CHAPTER 7:

Smoothie Recipes

20.   Green Mango Smoothie

Preparation Time: 5 Minutes

Cooking Time: 0 minutes

Servings: 1

Ingredients:

- 2 Cups Spinach

- 1-2 Cups Coconut Water

- 2 Mangos, Ripe, Peeled & Diced

Directions:

1. Blend everything together until smooth.

Nutrition: calories 120, fat 1, carbs 5, protein 8

21.   Chia Seed Smoothie

Preparation Time: 5 Minutes

Cooking Time: 0 minutes

Servings: 3

Ingredients:

- ¼ Teaspoon Cinnamon

- 1 Tablespoon Ginger, Fresh & Grated

- Pinch Cardamom

- 1 Tablespoon Chia Seeds

- 2 Medjool Dates, Pitted

- 1 Cup Alfalfa Sprouts

- 1 Cup Water

- 1 Banana

- ½ Cup Coconut Milk, Unsweetened

Directions:

1. Blend everything together until smooth.

Nutrition:

Calories: 412   Protein: 18.9g

Carbs: 43.8gFat: 24.8g

22.   Mango Smoothie

Preparation Time: 5 Minutes

Cooking Time: 0 minutes

Servings: 3

Ingredients:

- 1 Carrot, Peeled & Chopped

- 1 Cup Strawberries

- 1 Cup Water 1 Cup Peaches, Chopped

- 1 Banana, Frozen & sliced 1 Cup Mango, Chopped

Directions:

1. Blend everything together until smooth.

Nutrition: calories 221, fat 1, carbs 5, protein 4

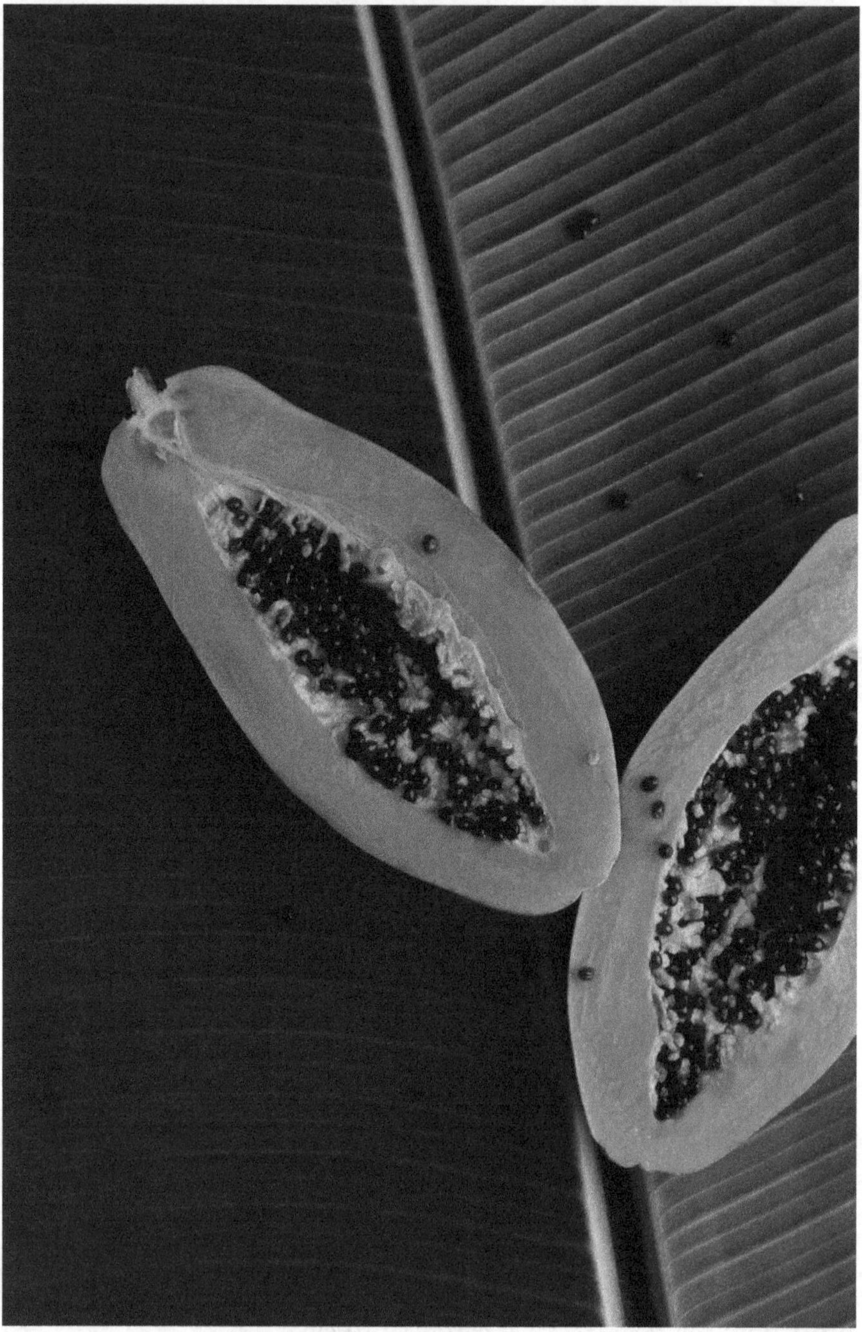

CHAPTER 8:

Fish and Seafood Recipes

23.   Savory Cilantro Salmon

Preparation Time: 10 minutes **Cooking Time:** 30 minutes

Servings: 4

Ingredients:

2 tablespoons of fresh lime or lemon

4 cups of fresh cilantro, divided

2 tablespoon of hot red pepper sauce

½ teaspoon of salt. Divided

1 teaspoon of cumin

4, 7 oz. of salmon filets

½ cup of (4 oz.) water

2 cups of sliced red bell pepper

2 cups of sliced yellow bell pepper

2 cups of sliced green bell pepper

Cooking spray ½ teaspoon of pepper

Directions:

Get a blender or food processor and combine half of the cilantro, lime juice or lemon, cumin, hot red pepper sauce, water, and salt; then puree until they become smooth. Transfer the marinade gotten into a large re-sealable plastic bag.

Add salmon to marinade. Seal the bag, squeeze out air that might have been trapped inside, turn to coat salmon. Refrigerate for about 1 hour, turning as often as possible.

Now, after marinating, preheat your oven to about 4000F. Arrange the pepper slices in a single layer in a slightly-greased, medium-sized square baking dish. Bake it for 20 minutes, turn the pepper slices once.

Drain your salmon and do away with the marinade. Crust the upper part of the salmon with the remaining chopped, fresh cilantro. Place salmon on the top of the pepper slices and bake for about 12-14 minutes until you observe that the fish flakes easily when it is being tested with a fork

Enjoy

Nutrition: Calories: 350 Carbohydrate: 15 g Protein: 42 g

Fat: 13 g

24. Cajun Catfish

Preparation Time: 10 minutes

Cooking Time: 10 minutes

Servings: 4

Ingredients:

- 16 oz catfish steaks (4 oz each fish steak)

- 1 tablespoon cajun spices

- 1 egg, beaten

- 1 tablespoon sunflower oil

Directions:

1. Pour sunflower oil into the skillet and preheat it until shimmering.

2. Meanwhile, dip every catfish steak in the beaten egg and coat it in Cajun spices.

3. Place the fish steaks in the hot oil and roast them for 4 minutes from each side.

4. The cooked catfish steaks should have a light brown crust.

Nutrition: calories 435, fat 7, carbs 8, protein 49

25.   4-Ingredients Salmon Fillet

Preparation Time: 5 minutes

Cooking Time: 25 minutes

Servings: 1

Ingredients:

- 4 oz salmon fillet

- ½ teaspoon salt

- 1 teaspoon sesame oil

- ½ teaspoon sage

Directions:

1. Rub the fillet with salt and sage.

2. Place the fish in the tray and sprinkle it with sesame oil.

3. Cook the fish for 25 minutes at 365F.

4. Flip the fish carefully onto another side after 12 minutes of

    cooking.

Nutrition: calories 190, fat 11, carbs 4, protein 22

26. Spanish Cod in Sauce

Preparation Time: 10 minutes

Cooking Time: 5.5 hours

Servings: 2

Ingredients*:*

- 1 teaspoon tomato paste

- 1 teaspoon garlic, diced

- 1 white onion, sliced

- 1 jalapeno pepper, chopped

- 1/3 cup chicken stock

- 7 oz Spanish cod fillet

- 1 teaspoon paprika

- 1 teaspoon salt

Directions:

1. Pour chicken stock into the saucepan.

2. Add tomato paste and mix up the liquid until homogenous.

3. Add garlic, onion, jalapeno pepper, paprika, and salt.

4. Bring the liquid to a boil and then simmer it.

5. Chop the cod fillet and add it to the tomato liquid.

6. Close the lid and simmer the fish for 10 minutes over low heat.

7. Serve the fish in the bowls with tomato sauce.

Nutrition: calories 112, fat 1, carbs 5, protein 18

27.   Fish Shakshuka

Preparation Time: 5 minutes

Cooking Time: 15 minutes

Servings: 5

Ingredients:

- 5 eggs

- 1 cup tomatoes, chopped 3 bell peppers, chopped

- 1 tablespoon butter

- 1 teaspoon tomato paste

- 1 teaspoon chili pepper

- 1 teaspoon salt

- 1 tablespoon fresh dill

- 5 oz cod fillet, chopped

- 1 tablespoon scallions, chopped

Directions:

1. Melt butter in the skillet and add chili pepper, bell peppers, and tomatoes.

2. Sprinkle the vegetables with scallions, dill, salt, and chili pepper. Simmer them for 5 minutes.

3. After this, add chopped cod fillet and mix up well.

4. Close the lid and simmer the ingredients for 5 minutes over medium heat.

5. Then crack the eggs over the fish and close the lid. Cook shakshuka with the closed lid for 5 minutes.

Nutrition: calories 143, fat 3, carbs 8, protein 12

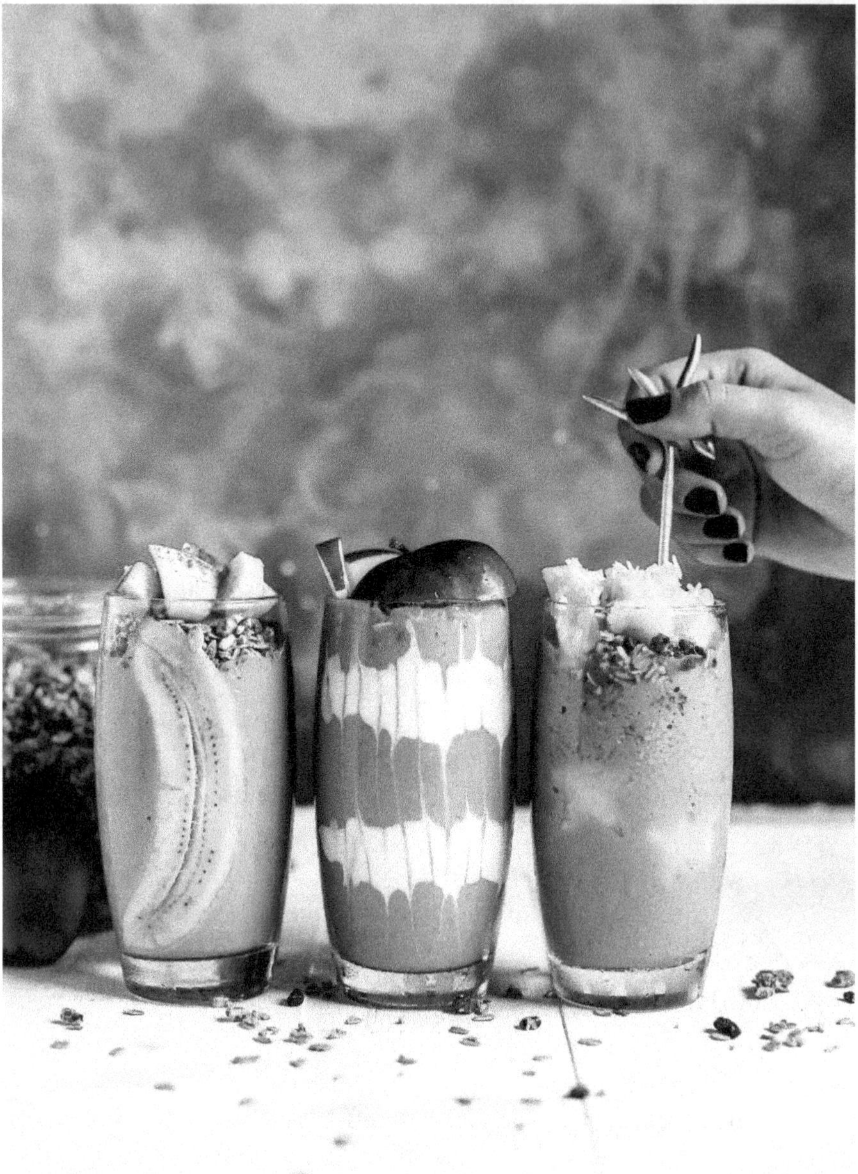

CHAPTER 9:

Poultry Recipes

28.   Chicken Fajita Roll Ups

Preparation time: 25 minutes

Cooking Time: 12 minutes

Servings: 6

Ingredients:

- 3 chicken breasts

- 1/2 red, green, and yellow bell pepper

- 1/2 red onion

- 2 teaspoons paprika

- 1 teaspoon garlic powder

- 1 teaspoon cumin powder

- 1/2 teaspoon cayenne

- 1/2 teaspoon oregano

- Salt and pepper, to taste

- Cooking spray

- Toothpicks

Directions:

1. Cut the bell pepper halves vertically into thin strips.

2. Mix together all of your spices.

3. Cut into half each chicken breast through the middle.

4. Pound each breast half flat.

5. Season both sides of each piece of chicken with the spice blend.

6. Place 2 bell pepper strips of each color and a few pieces of onion in the center of each piece of chicken.

7. Roll the chicken up around the peppers and onions and use 1 or 2 toothpicks to hold the roll up shut.

8. Preheat your air fryer to 390°F.

9. Spray each roll up with cooking spray and cook 3 at a time for 12 minutes.

Nutrition: Calories: 70, Fat: 2, Carbs: 3, Protein: 11

29.   Tandoori Chicken

Preparation time: 25 minutes

Cooking Time: 30 minutes

Servings: 4

Ingredients:

- 4 chicken legs

- 3 teaspoons ginger paste

- 3 teaspoons garlic paste

- Salt to taste

- 3 tablespoons lemon juice

- 2 tablespoon tandoori masala powder

- 1 teaspoon roasted cumin powder

- 1 teaspoon garam masala powder

- 2 teaspoons red chili powder

- 1 teaspoon turmeric powder

- 4 tablespoons hung curd

- 2 teaspoons kasoori methi

- 1 teaspoon black pepper

- 2 teaspoons coriander powder

Directions:

1. Wash the chicken legs and cut a few slits in each one. Mix ginger paste, garlic paste, and salt together.

2. Put the chicken in a bowl and coat with the ginger paste mix. Set the chicken in the fridge for 15 minutes.

3. While the chicken marinates, mix all the other ingredients together.

4. Pour the marinade over the chicken and return to the fridge for at least 10 hours.

5. Preheat the air fryer to 360°F. Cook the chicken for 30 minutes, turning halfway through.

Nutrition: Calories: 186, Fat: 12, Carbs: 5, Protein: 13

30.   Crispy Coconut Chicken

Preparation time: 15 minutes

Cooking Time: 15 minutes

Servings: 4

Ingredients:

- 1/2 cup cornstarch

- 1/4 Tbs. salt

- 1/8 teaspoon pepper

- 3 eggs

- 2 cups sweetened coconut flakes

- 2 cups unsweetened coconut flakes

- 4 medium boneless chicken breasts

Directions:

1. Beat the eggs and cut the chicken into strips.

2. Mix cornstarch, salt, and pepper in a separate bowl.

3. Place your sweetened and unsweetened coconut in a third shallow bowl or plate; mix well.

4. Roll the chicken in the cornstarch mix.

5. Dip the chicken in the egg, then roll it in coconut.

6. Preheat the air fryer to 360°F.

7. Cook for 15 minutes, flipping halfway through.

Nutrition: Calories: 452, Fat: 30, Carbs: 27, Protein: 19

31. Homemade Chicken Nuggets

Preparation time: 10 minutes

Cooking Time: 10 minutes

Servings: 4

Ingredients:

- 2 (8 ounce) skinless boneless chicken breasts, cut into nugget sized pieces

- Salt and pepper, to taste

- 2 teaspoons olive oil

- 6 tablespoons Italian seasoned breadcrumbs

- 2 tablespoons panko breadcrumbs

- 2 tablespoons parmesan cheese

- Olive oil spray

Directions:

1. Put chicken, olive oil, salt, and pepper in a bowl and toss to coat.

2. Mix the breadcrumbs and parmesan together in a bowl.

3. Toss the chicken in the breadcrumb mixture.

4. Place the chicken in the basket and spray with olive oil spray.

5. Preheat the air fryer to 390°F.

6. Cook for 10 minutes, tossing halfway through.

Nutrition: Calories: 338, Fat: 9, Carbs: 9, Protein: 50

CHAPTER 10:

Vegan & Vegetarian

32.   Healthy Vegetable Sauté

Preparation time: 15 minutes

Cooking Time: 16 minutes

Servings: 3

Ingredients:

- 2 tablespoons extra virgin olive oil

- 1 tablespoon minced garlic

- 1 large shallot, sliced

- 1 cup mushrooms, sliced

- 1 cup broccoli florets

- 1 cup artichoke hearts

- 1 bunch asparagus, sliced into 3-inch pieces

- 1 cup baby peas

- 1 cup cherry tomatoes, halved

- 1/2 teaspoon sea salt

- **Vinaigrette**

- 3 tablespoons white wine vinegar

- 6 tablespoons extra-virgin olive oil

- 1/2 teaspoon sea salt

- 1 teaspoon ground oregano

- Handful fresh parsley, chopped

Directions:

1. Add oil to the pan of your air fryer toast oven set over medium heat. Stir in garlic and shallots and sauté for about 2 minutes.

2. Stir in mushrooms for about 3 minutes or until golden.

3. Stir in broccoli, artichokes, and asparagus and continue cooking for 3 more minutes. Stir in peas, tomatoes, and salt and transfer to the air fryer toast oven and cook for 5-8 more minutes.

4. Prepare vinaigrette: mix together vinegar, oil, salt, oregano, and parsley in a bowl until well combined.

5. Serve vegetable sauté in a serving bowl and drizzle with vinaigrette.

6. Toss to combine and serve.

Nutrition: Calories 293, Fat 27, Carbs 14, Protein 25

33. Satisfying Grilled Mushrooms

Preparation time: 13 minutes

Cooking Time: 11 minutes

Servings: 4

Ingredients:

- 2 cups shiitake mushrooms

- 1 tablespoon balsamic vinegar

- 1/4 cup extra virgin olive oil 1-2 garlic cloves, minced

- A handful of parsley 1 teaspoon salt

Directions:

1. Rinse the mushroom and pat dry; put in a foil and drizzle with balsamic vinegar and extra virgin olive oil.

2. Sprinkle the mushroom with garlic, parsley, and salt.

3. Grill for about 10 minutes in your air fryer toast oven at 350 degrees F or until tender and cooked through.

4. Serve warm.

Nutrition: Calories 260, Fat 19, Carbs 11, Protein 22

34. Squash Pappardelle with Ricotta and Dried Tomato Sauce

Preparation time: 5 minutes

Cooking Time: 20 minutes

Servings: 4

Ingredients:

- 3 zucchini (ends trimmed)

- 3 medium squash (ends trimmed)

- 1 tsp. olive oil

- ½ tsp. salt

- Black pepper to taste

- ¼ cup sun-dried tomatoes (soaked in hot water for 10 minutes and drained)

- 1 tomato (seeded and coarsely chopped)

- 1 red bell pepper (halved and coarsely chopped)

- 1 garlic clove (minced) 1 tbsp. white balsamic vinegar

- 1 tbsp. olive oil ½ small shallot (diced)

- 12 fresh basil leaves (chopped)

- 1 cup ricotta cheese (part-skim)

Directions:

1. With a vegetable peeler, slice the zucchini and the squash lengthwise into paper-thin strips, then stack the strips and slice lengthwise to make ribbons (½ - inch thin).

2. Place the strips in a bowl and drizzle with oil, salt, black pepper, and sent them on the side to soften.

3. Meanwhile, put the drained sun-dried tomatoes in a food processor and blend for a few minutes to coarsely chop.

4. Add the fresh tomato, bell pepper, garlic, vinegar, and blend for a few minutes until just combined. While blending everything, slowly stream in oil, being careful not to over-process the mixture, since the sauce should be thick and a bit chunky.

5. Then, transfer to a bowl and fold in the red pepper flakes, shallot, and basil.

6. Serve.

Nutrition: Calories: 387 Fat: 6 g Carbohydrate: 14 gProtein: 18 g

35.   Mini Pepper Nachos

Cooking time: 20 minutes

Preparation time: 20 minutes

Servings: 4 servings

Ingredients:

- ¼ cup jalapeño (diced)

- Cooking spray

- 1,12 oz. can chicken (in water) drained

- 6 oz. avocado (mashed)

- ½ cup Greek yogurt

- 2 cups shredded cheddar cheese (low- fat, divided)

- 1 tsp. chili powder

- 24 mini bell peppers (halved, remove stem, seeds, and membranes)

- ¼ cup scallions (chopped)

Directions:

1. In a lightly greased pan, sauté the jalapeño until tender.

2. In a bowl, mix the jalapeño, chicken, avocado, Greek yogurt, one cup of cheddar cheese, and chili powder.

3. Put the mini bell peppers in a single layer in a casserole dish. Fill with chicken mixture, sprinkle with the remaining cheese, and broil until cheese has melted (about 2-4 minutes).

4. Garnish with scallions and serve with salsa, if desired.

Nutrition: Calories: 132 Carbs: 21g Fat: 4g Protein: 3g

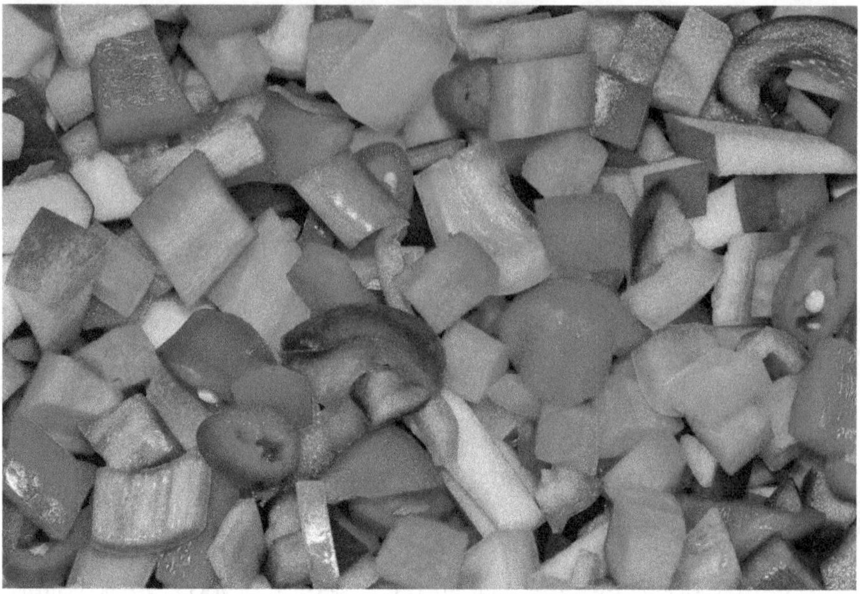

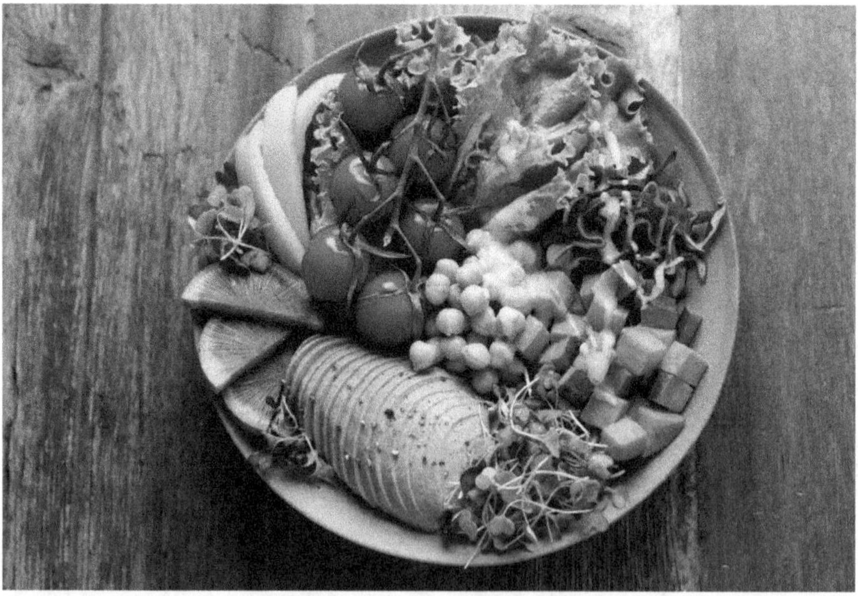

CHAPTER 11:

Pork recipes

36.   Panko Crusted Pork Chops

Preparation Time: 10 minutes

Cooking Time: 22 minutes

Servings: 2

Ingredients

- 1/4 tsp. salt

- 1/4 tsp. pepper

- 4 Boneless Pork chops

- 1 egg beaten

- 1 tbsp. Parmesan cheese

- 1 cup panko

- 1/2 tsp. granulated garlic

- 1/2 tsp. paprika

- 1/2 tsp. onion powder

- 1/2 tsp. chili powder

Directions

1. Preheat the air fryer toaster oven to 400 degrees while you prepare the pork chops. Spritz pork chops with salt on both sides and let it sit while you are preparing the seasonings and egg

wash. Put the beaten egg in a bowl. Flip the pork chops over

after 6 minutes if needed, spray with more olive oil spray and

keep cooking for the remaining 6 minutes.

Nutrition: Calories: 220, Fat: 6, Protein: 27, Carbs: 13

37.   Southern Style Pork Chops

Preparation Time: 10 minutes

Cooking Time: 25 minutes

Servings: 4

Ingredients

- 3 tbsp. buttermilk

- 4 pork chops

- Seasoning Salt to taste

- 1/4 cup flour

- Pork Seasoning

- 1 Ziploc bag

- Cooking oil spray

- Pepper to taste

Directions

1. Wash the pork chops and pat dry them. With the seasoning salt and pepper, season the pork chops. Pour the buttermilk over the pork chops. Put the pork chops in a Ziploc baggie with flour. Shake it to coat it completely. Marinate it for 30 minutes. Put the pork chops in the air fryer toaster oven. Spray the pork chops with cooking oil spray. Cook the pork chops at 380 degrees for 15 minutes. Turn the pork chops over to the other side after 10 minutes.

Nutrition: Calories: 173, Fat: 6, Protein: 22, Carbs: 7,

38. Damn Best Pork Chops

Preparation Time: 05 minutes

Cooking Time: 17 minutes

Servings: 2

Ingredients

- 2 Pork chops

- 1 1/2 tsp. salt

- 2 tbsp. brown sugar

- 1 tbsp. paprika

- 1 1/2 tsp. black pepper

- 2 tbsp. olive oil

- 1 tsp. ground mustard

- 1/2 tsp. onion powder

- 1/4 tsp. garlic powder

Directions

1. Preheat air fryer toaster oven to 400 degrees for 5 minutes. Wash pork chops with cool water and pat dry completely with a paper towel. In a bowl, add all the dry ingredients. Coat the pork chops with olive oil and brush in the mix. Brush it in well and liberally. Use all of the brushed mix for the 2 pork chops. Cook pork chops in air fryer toaster oven at 400 degrees for 12 minutes, turning pork chops over after 6 minutes if needed.

Nutrition: Calories: 198, Fat: 6g, Protein: 25g, Carbs: 10g, Fiber: 0g

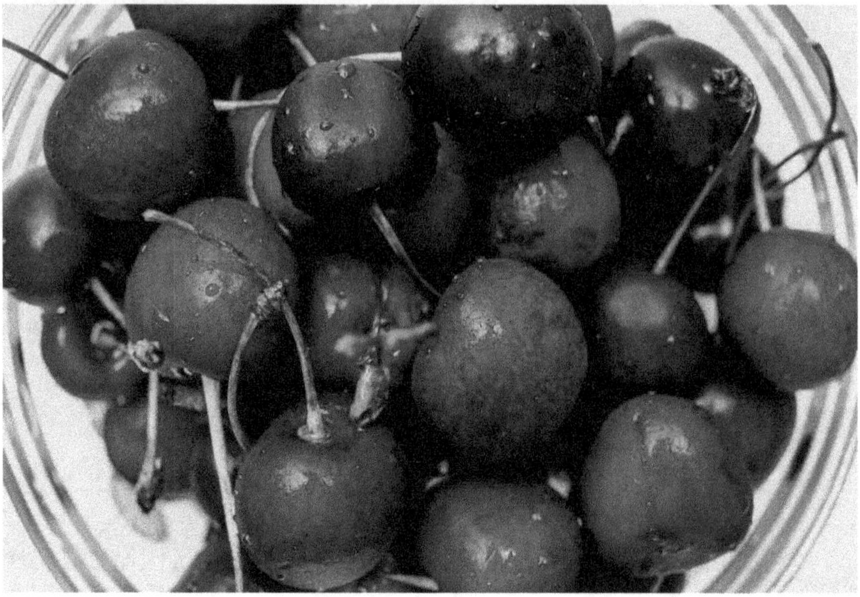

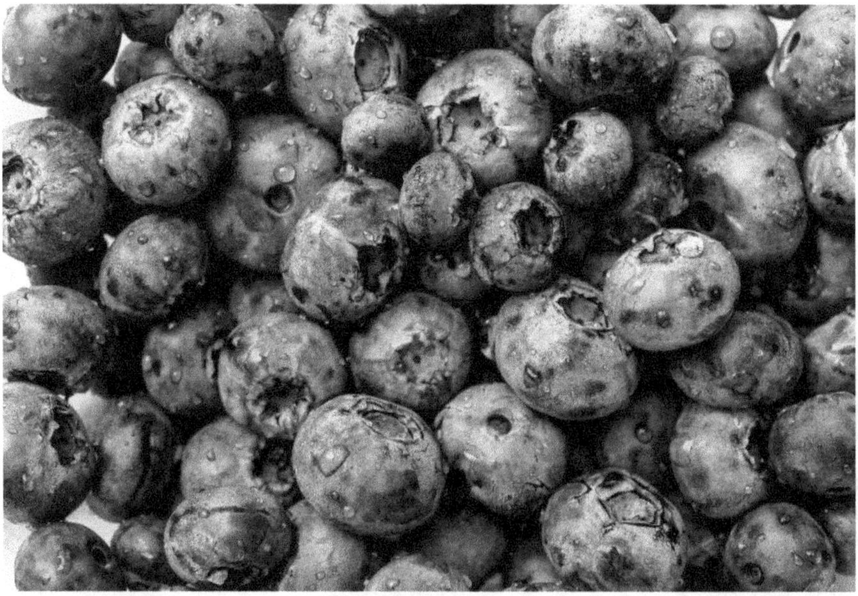

CHAPTER 12:

Snack Recipes

39.   Almond-Stuffed Dates

Preparation Time: 5 minutes

Cooking Time: 3 minutes

Servings: 4

Ingredients:

- 20 raw almonds

- 20 pitted dates

Directions:

1. Stuffed one almond into each of 20 dates. Serve at room temperature.

Nutrition: calories 223, fat 12, carbs 4, protein 12

CHAPTER 13:

Appetizer Recipes

40.   Greek Baklava

Preparation Time: *20 minutes* **Cooking Time**: *20 minutes*

Servings: 18

Ingredients:

- 1 (16 oz.) package phyllo dough

- 1 lb. chopped nuts

- 1 cup butter

- 1 teaspoon ground cinnamon

- 1 cup water

- 1 cup white sugar

- 1 teaspoon. vanilla extract

- 1/2 cup honey

Directions:

1. Preheat the oven to 175°C or 350°Fahrenheit. Spread butter on

    the sides and bottom of a 9-in by 13-in pan.

2. Chop the nuts, then mix with cinnamon; set it aside. Unfurl the

    phyllo dough, then halve the whole stack to fit the pan. Use a

    damp cloth to cover the phyllo to prevent drying as you proceed.

    Put two phyllo sheets in the pan, then butter well. Repeat to

    make eight layered phyllo sheets. Scatter 2-3 tablespoons. nut mixture over the sheets, then place two more phyllo sheets on top, butter, then sprinkle with nuts. Layer as you go. The final layer should be six to eight phyllo sheets deep.

3. Make square or diamond shapes with a sharp knife up to the bottom of the pan. You can slice into four long rows for diagonal shapes. Bake until crisp and golden for 50 minutes.

4. Meanwhile, boil water and sugar until the sugar melts to make the sauce; mix in honey and vanilla. Let it simmer for 20 minutes.

5. Take the baklava out of the oven, then drizzle with sauce right away; cool. Serve the baklava in cupcake papers. You can also freeze them without cover. The baklava will turn soggy when wrapped.

Nutrition: Calories: 255 Fat: 15g   Saturated Fat: 4g   Trans Fat: 0g

Cholesterol: 14g   Fiber: 2g   Sodium: 403mg Protein: 25g

Conclusion

When you desire a structure and need to rapidly lose weight, the present diet is the perfect solution.

Its extremely low calories eating plans of the optavia diet will definitely help you to shed more pounds

Before you start any meal replacement diet plan, carefully consider if truly it possible for you to continue with a specific diet plan

When you have decided to stick with this regimen and make progress with your weight loss goal, ensure you have a brilliant knowledge about optimal health management to enable and archive the desired result effortlessly in the shortest period of time.

CPSIA information can be obtained
at www.ICGtesting.com
Printed in the USA
LVHW081327220621
690776LV00010B/489